Battling Burnout

Strategies for Overcoming Debilitating Stress and Reclaiming Your Best Life

Anthony Glenn

Table of Contents

What is Burnout?

If you are constantly stressed, overwhelmed, and exhausted, you find it hard to get out of bed, you feel you're not appreciated, and there's no hope anything will change, there's no point in going to work, and all effort is useless, you are probably experiencing burnout. This is a state of physical, mental, and emotional exhaustion caused by prolonged and excessive stress. Burnout provokes extreme fatigue; you feel drained and that you have nothing more to give. It can cause serious damage to your work, relationships, and health. When you are unable to meet constant demands, you lose interest and motivation, start to question your ability, and your energy fades. It reduces your productivity and you are left hopeless, helpless, and full of resentment. The negative effects of burnout spread to all areas of life—your career, your home life, relationships, health, and social life. It also causes changes to your body, making you vulnerable to illnesses from colds and the flu, to more serious conditions.

Burnout can hit anyone who is constantly exposed to high stress, including businesspeople, CEOs, students, stay-at-home-moms, and anyone overloaded with invisible work and taking care of others. On the other hand, not everyone exposed to stress will develop this condition. If stress is well-managed, it may not do any damage.

Signs and Symptoms

We all have days when dragging ourselves out of bed is particularly hard, especially when we feel overloaded and unappreciated. But if you feel like this most of the time and every day is a bad day for you, you may be burned out.

Burnout doesn't happen overnight. It is a gradual process. The signs and symptoms are not too obvious at first, but become worse as time goes on. The early, subtle symptoms are red flags that something is wrong and you need to change something. If you pay attention, address the problem, and do everything to reduce your stress, you can prevent a colossal breakdown. But if you ignore them, you'll eventually burn out.

Symptoms that signal something's wrong and that you might be on the path to burnout are many, and include physical, emotional, and behavioral clues. Here are some of them.

- Frequent headaches or muscle pain
- Feeling tired most of the time
- Loss of motivation
- Lowered immunity, frequent illnesses
- Change in appetite or sleep habits
- Feeling helpless, trapped, and defeated
- Decreased satisfaction and sense of accomplishment
- Procrastinating, taking longer to get things done

- Taking out your frustrations on others
- Sense of failure and self-doubt
- Detachment, feeling alone in the world
- An increasingly cynical and negative outlook
- Using food, drugs, or alcohol to cope
- Skipping work, coming in late, or leaving early
- Withdrawing from responsibilities
- Isolating yourself from others

It's Not Just Stress

Unrelenting stress may lead to burnout, but it's not the same thing. Stress demands a majority of your energy and effort; it exerts too much pressure to meet too many demands. However, stressed people know that everything can still be fine if just they manage to get things under control.

On the other hand, being burned out means that you don't have enough energy, you lack motivation, feel empty and drained, and see no hope of change. While stressed people are aware that they are drowning in responsibilities, you're not always aware of burnout when it's happening.

While stress is characterized by over-engaging, with burnout, you don't feel like engaging anymore. Emotions are overactive while you are stressed, but with burnout, they are blunted. Stressed people often feel urgency and hyperactivity. Conversely, people who are going through burnout often feel helpless and hopeless. In stress, you lack energy. In burnout, you lack even more—motivation and hope. If you do nothing to resolve it, stress will lead you to an anxiety disorder. Burnout, on the other hand, leads to depression. The primary damage that stress produces is physical; the damage caused by burnout is emotional. While stress may kill you prematurely, burnout will make you question if life is worth living.

Causes of Burnout

Leading causes of burnout may stem from your job, but that's not the only possible source. A stressful job doesn't have to provoke burnout. If it's handled well, everything will be fine. Anyone who feels overworked and undervalued is vulnerable to burnout, from a bartender who hasn't had a vacation in years, to the housewife who feels no one appreciates her work.

Burnout is not only caused by overlong to-do lists and stressful work. Other factors, including your personality traits and lifestyle, contribute to burnout. In fact, how you look at the world and what you do in your leisure time has a big role in causing stress. It's not solely about overwhelming stress at work or home.

Work-related causes of burnout

- Feeling like you have little control over your work or feeling that you have no control over your circumstances in any field is a source of permanent stress and exhaustion.
- Lack of recognition and reward: Feeling underappreciated for good work is disappointing. No one is motivated to put more effort into something that no one else recognizes.
- Lack of support and communication with a manager, a team leader, or an employer.
- Unclear or overly demanding job expectations: Only 60% of workers know what is expected of them. When expectations are constantly changing, employees may become exhausted

simply by trying to figure out what they are supposed to be doing.

- Unreasonable time pressure: Employees who are not able to gain more time for their tasks, like firefighters or paramedics, are at a high risk of burnout. Workers who have enough time for their work don't have this problem.
- Doing work that's monotonous or unchallenging: You can't maintain excitement about something unexciting. If there's no challenge, you are not motivated to perform your best.
- Working in a chaotic or high-pressure environment: Human beings need some level of order and peace. If you are under constant pressure, it's just a matter of time before you break down.
- Unmanageable workload: Even the most optimistic employees will lose hope and motivation if a workload feels unmanageable. Being overwhelmed undoubtedly leads to burnout.
- Unfair treatment: Whether it's favoritism, unfair compensation, or poor relationships with co-workers, employees who are treated unfairly are more likely to experience burnout.

Lifestyle causes of burnout

- Not getting enough sleep: If you constantly lack sleep, you can't run away from exhaustion and it will creep up on you sooner or later.
- Working too much without enough free time for relaxing: The key ingredient against burnout is balance. You need all areas of your life to

achieve balance; otherwise, you are at risk of burnout.
- Lack of close, supportive relationships: Strong, positive relationships with people who are close to you are crucial for happiness and fulfillment. Without them, you are more exposed to stress and exhaustion.
- Taking on too many responsibilities without help from others: You cannot and should not handle life on your own. Asking for help is never a sign of weakness.

Personality traits that contribute to burnout

- Perfectionism: If you believe nothing is ever good enough and you need to do whatever possible to make it as close to perfection as you can, that's the recipe for exhaustion. Things will still be imperfect and you'll also be burned out.
- Pessimism: Looking at the world and yourself through negative lenses is exhausting. If you pair it with stress, it's a perfect combination for burnout.
- The need to be in control and hesitate to delegate to others: If you think that you have to do everything on your own if you want it done right, you are likely to experience exhaustion.
- High-achieving, Type A personality: If you are always focused on achievement instead of the process, that's difficult. Chances are that you simply don't know how to relax and do nothing.

How to Recover from Burnout

Once you realize that you're going through burnout, you've made a first step towards overcoming it. But simply being aware of what's going on won't solve your problem. Exhaustion won't resolve itself. You need to do something about it, and simply getting more sleep is not the ultimate cure. Of course, sleep is one of the key factors in recovery, but not the only one. Here are some things you can do to help yourself recover and overcome this condition. (You can call it a phase, a problem, a bad time. We'll call it a condition.)

Before anything else, stop doing what you do

Stop the project, pause, take a break, go on vacation. Give yourself some time off to recharge. Doing the same thing over again won't give you results that are any different from those you've already gotten. Ask yourself what can wait. (What can I cancel? Which tasks can I put on a waitlist?) Probably some of your tasks can be postponed. Ask your boss or a supervisor, employer, or clients to extend deadlines. Ask which projects can wait and which are urgent. Perhaps you can't cancel all of your duties (especially if you are a parent, for instance), but there's always something you can put off. Maybe it's an evening out, a social event, some extra activity, or a chore that doesn't have to be done right now. Decide to give yourself and your health the priority. Everything else can wait. You might be surprised by the fact that the world won't stop spinning.

Focus on the basics

You need to say "no" to all unnecessary events and projects so you can say "yes" to your well-being. For recharging your battery, it's crucial to focus only on the basics. We are talking about your most elementary needs: sleep, food, and water.

"But that's so unproductive!" your mind is protesting. We are so trained to strive for productivity that we have a hard time accepting that it is not our only purpose.

You don't need to be productive now. You need to recover from burnout. Striving to be as productive as possible and neglecting your essential needs brought you here. Now it's time to do the opposite and take more care of yourself.

Sleep

Although getting more sleep by itself is not enough to overcome exhaustion, it's one of the fundamental factors in beating it. The World Health Organization recommends seven to nine hours of sleep a day. However, more than 40% of the population sleeps less than seven hours. Scientific research has shown that our brain suffers if we lack sleep. Our prefrontal cortex shrinks, the part responsible for reasoning, planning, and memory. During sleep, our body and mind resolves any small issues that appear during the day, and can recharge and rejuvenate. If you don't afford that to yourself, it can lead to many health issues and even premature death. From this point of view, burnout is not necessarily a bad thing—it's good to know when you are drained. Your body and mind are doing their best to stop you and force you to rest.

Saying that you don't have much time for sleep because you need to be more productive is the same as saying that you don't have time to stop at a gas station to fuel your vehicle.

So first of all, listen to this simple advice and really get more sleep. If you already suffer from insomnia, you might need to put some extra effort into this step. As well as sleeping more, you also need better quality sleep. Here is some advice on how to accomplish that:

1. Let yourself rest and recharge. Give yourself permission to leave everything alone for now.

Let the work stay where it belongs. Let everything go. Decide that it's time only to sleep and recharge. There's nothing you should be accomplishing now. Realize you are absolutely free from any obligations except resting your body and mind.

2. Unplug.

Turn off your phone, your computer, your laptop. Avoid watching TV before bed, and don't scroll through Facebook or Instagram. Everything you do before bed you take with you into sleep. You don't need all of that crap with you—no bad news or useless information. There's no need for you to be available to everyone all the time. It's best to turn your phone off or put it on airplane mode. The blue light that monitors emit wakes up your mind, which should be calm before sleep.

3. Go to bed early.

It would be best to be in bed before 10:00 p.m. That way, your mind and body will have enough time to recharge before midnight—certain processes in the brain happen only in that time frame. Sleeping two hours before midnight is not the same as getting two hours of sleep after midnight.

4. Try to go to bed always at the same time.

This is how you'll build a habit, and your body and mind will be prepared at the right time so you'll already be relaxed enough to fall asleep faster.

5. Relax before bedtime.

You can try to meditate, have a bubble bath, read a book, or do anything else that makes you relax and doesn't include screens and social networks.

6. Sleep in a dark room.

Turn off all the lights and pull thick curtains closed in order to dim street lights. You can also use a sleep mask. The thing is, it's only in the dark that our bodies produce certain chemicals responsible for restoring our cells and maintaining optimal health.

7. Let fresh air in.

This one is obvious. Because we spend a lot of time sleeping, it's important to inhale fresh air while you sleep. But besides that, letting fresh air into the room will help you fall asleep and have better quality sleep. Try to sleep with open windows, or if you that's not feasible, open all of them an hour or two before bedtime so you have a purified room when you go to bed.

8. Use lavender oil.

This aromatic oil has magnificent effects on our ability to relax and fall asleep. You can inhale it, pour some into your evening bath, or spray your pillow and bedsheets with it. There are also cosmetic products with lavender scent, so you could try those as well. Lighting a scented candle with this fragrance is also a good choice—just don't forget to blow it out before going to bed.

9. Listen to white noise.

It's been proven that listening to sounds of rain, the ocean, or any other kind of white noise helps us fall asleep. You can find numerous different types of these on YouTube or even invest in a white noise machine. It might require some time to adjust to this, but in a few nights you'll be sleeping like a baby.

10. Try a guided meditation.

Meditation is one of the best ways to relax. Ideally, you can completely relax the whole body, part by part, starting with your feet. Guided meditation is ideal for beginners because it helps focus your undivided attention on relaxing every inch of your body. A voice tells you what to do, and you just follow the instructions. Again, you can find many of them on YouTube. Just listen to a few to make sure you like the voice that will be leading you into relaxation. It can be pretty annoying if you don't like the voice while you are trying to relax.

11. Drink a cup of tea or a glass of warm milk.

There's something soothing in the ritual of sipping a warm liquid before bedtime, like having a warm bath.

There are some special kinds of tea, also known as sleepytime or bedtime teas. They are herbal, caffeine-free, and contain ingredients which are also used in sleep supplements.

Bedtime teas help create a calming bedtime experience by combining anti-anxiety and pro-sleep herbal ingredients. Some of them have sedative effects, while others fight insomnia by reducing stress and anxiety. The best-known are chamomile, valerian, lavender, lemon balm, spearmint, and catnip in the mint family. Although the effect of these teas is mild, the placebo effect should be enough to help you fall asleep.

The idea of drinking a glass of warm milk before bedtime for better sleep is quite old. Milk contains tryptophan, an amino acid that impacts serotonin and melatonin production, responsible for a person's sleep-wake cycle. Also, the calcium in milk can help a person stay asleep, so it's an effective natural sleep aid.

12. Choose the right pillows and mattress.

If there is something that your tomorrow-self will be grateful for to your today-self, it's choosing the proper support for your rest. Invest in a quality mattress and pillows, and you'll benefit in every area. It will help you overcome burnout, but also allow you to perform your best each day from now on.

Clean up your diet to help yourself recover from burnout

I know this one is not exciting at all, but it's crucial, alongside sleeping well and light workouts. What we put in our mouths is the first place to start healing and recovering from what our bodies have been through.

While we are going through a stressful period, most of us neglect our basic needs, including diet. We often grab the nearest source of fuel and just gulp it down to get the energy to make it through the day. You take in calories, but your body remains unnourished. This significantly contributes to overall exhaustion. When you want to undo the effects of such behavior, it's time to pay attention to what you put in your body.

1. Plan it.

If you don't want to switch back your old habits and just shove down Big Macs, you need a plan and a stock of healthy foods. It all requires some energy and effort, but it will pay off; otherwise, you will just go on feeling exhausted. You need to map out your diet, go to the grocery store to stock up, and plan your meals in advance. If you live a busy life (and who doesn't?), you may find it easier to make a weekly menu. Do the main shopping once a week and then stick to the plan on a daily basis. Make a weekly plan for breakfast, lunch, dinner, and don't forget to fit two snacks into the menu.

2. Trade large meals for smaller ones.

While recovering from exhaustion, you don't want a high oscillation of sugar levels. Eating large meals once or twice a day will do exactly that—torture your body with starving and sugar ups and downs.

Divide them into smaller portions and eat five to six times throughout the day. Don't even think about skipping any meals! Your body needs your care, so be gentle with your sugar levels. Ideally, try to eat your breakfast before 10:00 a.m, and don't punish your body with intermittent fasting. It's already tired enough.

3. Say no to coffee and caffeine, alcohol, smoking, and drugs.

"Not my coffee!" you're screaming. What's wrong with coffee? It's not the best warm drink for when you're going through burnout. It might overstimulate your body and mind, and worsen the symptoms of anxiety and depression, putting you into fight or flight mode. That's the opposite of what you want. Caffeine has that effect, which is why some people find it too stimulating if consumed late in the afternoon or evening. Others, however, show that caffeine has nothing to do with sleeping. Also, your doctor might tell you that one to two cups a day is fine. You need to find what works for you—you might want to keep your two coffees a day or cut it out completely, at least for a time.

When it comes to alcohol, smoking, and other substances, it's another story. Do your best to avoid them completely. Although it might be challenging, it's necessary for your recovery. Prioritize your health over those temporary, harmful satisfactions. Your body will be far happier.

4. Eliminate sugar from your diet.

This is the single most effective change any of us can make. Seriously, you will feel like a new person and your body will thank you. It's especially apparent when you are fighting adrenaline and sugar peaks and crashes. We are all so programmed to love sweets, that often it becomes a habit instead of a treat. Natural alternatives to processed sugar, like honey, are a much better choice, although they mess up sugar levels, too. Try to keep a supply of good alternatives like nuts, energy bars, and so on. Drinking a lot of water, especially lemon water, is great because we often mistake thirstiness for craving for sweets. Besides that, if it's in any way possible, take a nap because it's too easy to grab something sweet when you lack energy and need a little rest. Take little steps day by day, drink a lot of water, rest whenever possible, and you'll get rid of the bad habit.

5. Eliminate highly-processed foods; eat more wholefoods, fresh fruits, and veggies.

It's not enough to avoid pizza-flavored chips and other obvious chemical products. These days, almost everything packaged is likely to have too much salt and/or sugar in it.

The opposite of processed food is whole food—foods that are not processed, altered, or packed in layers of plastic. When you consume only or mainly that sort of food, you feel much lighter, fresher, and more energized.

Eat more fresh fruits and veggies, nuts and seeds, natural oils, organic meat if you consume meat, eggs, fish, and whole grains. The options are numerous. Keep in mind that it's best to cook your meals at home, and when it comes to fueling your body, quick fixes are usually the worst.

6. Cut down on inflammatory foods.

When it comes to cleaning out your diet, you might also want to cut down on inflammatory foods, such as dairy and gluten. A huge number of people are intolerant to these things, but not aware of it. They may provoke gastrointestinal issues and irritations that send signals to our nervous system to trigger mood changes.

7. Ingest more omega-3 fatty acids.

Since the human brain is about 60% fat, it's essential to eat enough healthy fats. Fat fish is rich in omega-3 acids, which are linked to decreasing depression and anxiety symptoms, and overall mood increases. Eating healthy fats helps our body to absorb vitamins and antioxidants from fat, and keep our sugar levels stable. They significantly reduce anxiety and depression, which contributes to burnout. So try to eat some healthy fats with each meal and at least three servings of fatty fish a week.

8. Soups and smoothies

Soups, warm beverages, and smoothies are all comforting, delicious, and incredibly healthy. These are easy ways to squeeze in a lot of nutrients, antioxidants, healthy fats, and fiber and make a delicious meal. You can make a soup from fiber-rich vegetables, add a topping of healthy oil, and even add some protein, making it a complete meal. Smoothies are an excellent way to blend together many vegetables and fruits you would never consume otherwise. You can add healthy fats, boosters like goji berries, maca, bee pollen, or additional proteins to your smoothie and boost its nutritional value.

9. Supplements

Although there is no magic pill or quick fix for extreme fatigue, exhaustion, and burnout, there is some additional aid for a speedy recovery. Pumping your body full of vital nutrients will surely help. Here are some supplements you can try (some or all of them). It would be best to take them daily for at least the first four to six weeks of your recovery.

- Magnesium bisglycinate (take 450-600 mg per day)
- Ashwagandha
- Zinc
- Liposomal vitamin C
- Omega 3 + DHA
- B vitamin complex
- Caffeine-free electrolyte tablets
- Liposomal glutathione
- Holy basil tincture
- Licorice root extract

- Flaxseed oil
- A high quality, organic greens powder

A workout for burnout recovery

We all know how super-important it is to keep moving. When you are healthy, you should exercise to maintain health. When you have a health issue, moving will probably be on the list of things you should follow. If you are pregnant or you are recovering from giving birth or surgery, guess what? You need to work out!

When you are super-busy, you perhaps skip your workout routine. But when you are trying to undo the bad effects of burnout, your body needs movement. You need to develop a new exercise routine that will serve you throughout this period.

I know, it's easier said than done. When you don't even want to leave your bed in the morning, you might not want to go to the gym where a personal trainer will kick your butt. But you still have to find the proper way to make your body move.

Exercise has a well-known anti-stress effect. Moderate exercise produces mood-elevating neurotransmitters, including endorphins, dopamine, serotonin, and norepinephrine. The movement also breaks down stress hormones, so you can relax more easily.

However, for those who are truly exhausted, moderation is crucial. If you are pushing yourself too hard, you'll just add more stress to your overall adrenal fatigue and it can be just as harmful as a sedentary lifestyle, triggering your fight-or-flight response with attendant surges of cortisol.

That's why cardio is not a good choice for you right now. When you're chronically stressed or suffering from adrenal fatigue, extreme cardio and intense workouts can actually cause you to gain weight.

When your already-elevated cortisol levels due to chronic stress combine with the cortisol spikes of daily cardio sessions, you're essentially creating a "fat trap." Your body thinks you're in fight-or-flight mode constantly. In response, it holds on to extra calories and stores fuel as body fat (especially around your midsection)—a good thing when you're trying to survive in the desert; not so good when you live in the modern-day world.

Instead, practice some restorative exercises like yoga. Taking walks is also an excellent choice. You can also try a less intense variation of standard interval training, in which short sessions of intensive exercises are followed by periods of recovery. Alternating exertion with rest will trigger your body to relax through movement.

One more perfect way to exercise when burnt out is simple walking. Walking increases circulation, boosts metabolism, improves breathing, and clears the head, without pushing an already exhausted system too hard.

Keep in mind that if you find yourself even more tired the day after your workout, that's the signal that you may have been pushing a bit too hard. Whatever kind of exercise you engage in, make sure you aren't overexerting yourself.

Practicing yoga is one more perfect solution for the phase of imbalance you are going through. Find yoga classes in your neighborhood, or if you already have some experience with it, try to do it at home.

Yoga is a holistic practice, which means that it encompasses body, mind, and spirit. The practice of yoga can help to level out areas of your life where you have gotten off-balance. Yoga works to guide you through self-study and inquiry, to bring you on a path that is most suited to your needs. When you are going through a period of imbalance, some of your chakras (energy centers) and nadis (energy channels) might be over or under-stimulated. This inhibits or poorly directs the flow of prana (energy or life force) and can cause a sense of feeling stuck or stagnant. Practicing yoga will bring knowledge about it to the surface.

Yoga will bring you more self-awareness and quieting of the mind, so you'll be able to hear messages you previously couldn't hear from the background noise. You'll be able to notice the sources of your life imbalance and why you became burnt out in the first place. This will help you combat your sense of confusion by gaining more insights and better understanding. Once you learn to be more self-aware, it will prevent you from experiencing burnout again in the future, through noticing how you are living your daily life and making the appropriate adjustments for living a more balanced existence.

Hydration

Yes, we were serious when we said to focus on the basics, even something as basic as drinking water. "How could anyone forget to drink water?" you might ask.

One quite common sign of burnout is dehydration. As energy starts to fade, people reach for caffeine and energy drinks to keep it up. But although it keeps us awake, caffeine is a diuretic. Drinking beverages like coffee or green, white, or black teas are definitely not substitutes for water. Instead of refreshing and keeping you hydrated, they actually contribute to dehydration.

The general recommendations are eight 8 oz. glasses of water a day. Another way to discover your ideal water intake is to divide your weight (in pounds) by two. As a result, you'll get the number of ounces of water you need each day. For example, if you weigh 140 lbs., strive to drink 70 ounces of water daily.

If you are still not sure about this, you have a perfect navigating tool—your thirst! That is the most basic, natural way of telling us we need water.

If you are drinking enough water, your urine will show it. If it is clear or light yellow, you are well-hydrated. The more dehydrated you are, the darker the urine is.

You can make hydration more interesting and spruce it up with lemon, mint, other fruits or berries, but make sure you are drinking enough water.

Breathing

Can this be more crucial than drinking water? Yes, there is something even more fundamental—your breathing.

Learning how to breathe properly and to slow down is one of the biggest tools for well-being that you can give yourself.

If you knew your breathing had a direct impact on your ability to manage stress, you would have paid more attention to it.

Place your hand on your chest and the other on your belly. Now breathe, and notice which one is moving more. If it's the one on your belly, congratulations, you are doing it right. But if you are like most of us, your breath is rapid, shallow, and high in your chest.

Breathing this way day in, day out activates your sympathetic nervous system and triggers fight-or-flight mode. You are permanently switched on to stress.

Did you know that 70% of the waste that our bodies produce is removed by our breath?

Moreover, if we knew how to use our breath, we could use it to energize ourselves instead of using coffee or to help us sleep better than drinking a glass of wine. You can also use it to remain calm when stress levels become unbearable.

However, no one will ask you how are you breathing if you do tests and checks to figure out what's wrong with you.

Once you learn how to use all the power of your breath, your life will never be the same again, and burnout will be a thing of the past.

Learning to breathe like a child again, deeply and freely from your diaphragm and your belly instead high up in your chest, is a life skill and one of the biggest favors you can do for yourself.

Shallow breathing high in the chest provokes a stress reaction by activating the fight or flight response of our sympathetic nervous system. That's why you feel like you are in danger, although you're facing just another task on your to-do list.

Deep, slow breathing, on the other hand, activates our parasympathetic nervous system, responsible for the "rest and digest" mode.

Have you noticed that every emotion has a corresponding breath? Notice how your breathing changes in response to different life experiences. It's different in a stressful and challenging situation from the breathing you do while you are relaxed.

Once you are aware of it, you can begin to learn how to use your breath to support your health and well-being.

You can use it to consciously connect with yourself, to remain grounded and calm even in stressful times.

One of the most studied and researched of all the thousands of breathing techniques out there is the one called the 365 technique:

- 3 times a day
- 6 breaths a minute
- 5 minutes at a time

Sit comfortably upright with your back straight, and make sure your breathing is not restricted by your clothing.

Breathe in through your nose deeply to allow your belly to expand outward. Count to five.

Feel the breath slowly in waves up to your chest as your ribs expand.

Count of six while you're exhaling slowly through your nose. Feel your belly deflate like a balloon during the breath ripple in reverse, down through your chest into your diaphragm and ribs.

Repeat this breathing exercise for five minutes, three times a day.

In the morning, you can use it to balance your system before starting the day; in the afternoon, it can be used as a recovery for low energy levels. You can use it in the evening as a relaxation routine before bedtime. It's also a great technique for conquering anxiety.

You will feel calm and relaxed. It brings down cortisol levels, strengthens the immune system, and boosts authentic energy. It's like you hit the reset button to calm your nervous system.

Reach out for help

If you've hit rock bottom, you've likely been shouldering too much for a long time.

Perhaps you find it hard to ask for help. Maybe you believe that you have to do everything on your own if you want it to be done right. You might feel a lack of support, that no one has your back.

Stop trying to carry everything on your own. No one is strong enough to do it forever. Everyone will crash down sooner or later. It's not a sign of weakness to ask for help, to share the work, to delegate.

Let your close people in. Tell your family and friends that you are struggling and what you're going through. They will probably want to help if they only knew how much you needed help.

We are social beings. You are not an exception. Connect or reconnect with others. It's a powerful aid against depression, anxiety, and burnout. Life is nicer when you have others to rely on.

Find your healers

Yes, your family and friends are the most significant support for your recovery journey. But you should also enlist cures from professional healers.

It might be enough for you to visit your doctor to find out what's wrong with you and why you don't feel fine. But you may want to visit more healers with different approaches in order to rule out any possible health reasons for your condition and to get more opinions. It might be a medical doctor, a naturopath, a massage therapist, an acupuncturist, an energy healer, a psychotherapist, and many others. There are numerous alternative ways to heal, from homeopathy, to crystals, to yoga, and so on.

You won't find one magic pill to solve your problem. Lots of little things are going to add up to help you to heal.

Think about the "why" of burnout

Although the roots of extreme exhaustion are more or less the same, each of us has some particular things that have led to burnout. A bartender's burnout, the burnout of a yoga teacher, of a student, or stay-at-home mom have different causes.

What brought you here?

You need to identify why you're experiencing burnout. It might be obvious or you may have to dig deeper.

Do you feel any resentment towards your work? Usually, resentment is an indicator that something is wrong or missing.

For instance, you may love your job, but hate that you are missing precious time with your family. If your boss doesn't recognize that or even has more demands and never mentions how hard you work, you are likely to feel resentment. In this case, you don't experience burnout because you hate your job—you love it. But you hate missing out on time with your family and neglecting your personal life.

If you are a stay-at-home mom, it's not about not loving your kids enough. You are just drained of constantly repeating the same routine, without your purpose in sight. You might be missing some me-time, going out with your friends, alone time with your spouse, talking to someone grown-up, and other activities that don't include kids and the kitchen.

Use introspection to get to the root of the problem and find out what about your role is bothering you. Once you've come to the reason for your burnout, write down ways that come to mind about how you can manage or eliminate that source of stress or unhappiness.

To identify the underlying causes of burnout, you can keep a stress diary. Write down what made you feel stressed and why every day. That can give you deep insights. It's fine to write it down as long as you need to, in order to find root and manage stress.

Once you know what caused your burnout, see what you can do to resolve it. This might involve extreme changes like altering your role; or less extreme, like making some changes in your job, delegating some of your tasks to others, working from home, or something else.

Question your values and goals

A million little decisions led you to your particular form of burnout. But the root cause is the same—what you do is out of alignment with your values, or your work doesn't contribute to your long-term goal. Or you don't even have goals and don't know where you're going.

For instance, if you value financial gain over your family, don't be surprised your relationships with your family are not perfect. You need to know your priorities. Health, family, love, finances—everything should have its own place. But if you value finances over your health, sooner or later it's going to cause issues.

Take a moment to sit with the question, "What do I value the most?"

Think about how your values are incorporated into your work. What gives you a sense of meaning and purpose? What is your mission? What do you have and want to offer to the world? And what cost are you willing to pay? Every one of us has something valuable to offer to society, but not everyone is willing to do it at the cost of health or family.

This self-analysis will give you awareness and understanding of what's most important to you, and it will show you which elements are missing from your life or work.

After this period of introspection, see how you can incorporate your mission and values into your current role. This might mean crafting your job to fit better to your personality, or just changing the way you're looking at your role.

According to the PERMA model well-known in psychology, we all need five crucial elements in our lives to experience well-being. These are positive emotions, engagement, relationships, meaning, and achievement. Use this model for orientation and notice whether any of these elements are missing, and find ways to incorporate them into your life.

1. Positive emotions

We all need positive emotions to experience well-being. Satisfaction, pleasure, peace, gratitude, hope, inspiration, curiosity, love, they all fall into this category. It's important to enjoy yourself in the here and now, together with other elements of PERMA in their place.

2. Engagement

If you want to experience a state of flow, to stop time, forget about yourself, be completely in the present, be truly engaged in what you're doing. The more you experience complete engagement, the more well-being you'll experience.

3. Relationships

Humans are social beings, and relationships are at the heart of our well-being. People who have meaningful, positive relationships with others are far happier than those who don't.

4. Meaning

To have a sense of well-being, we all need meaning in our lives and feel that we serve a cause bigger than ourselves. This might be anything that serves humanity in some way.

5. Achievement

One more thing that contributes to our ability to enjoy life is an accomplishment. We all strive to better ourselves. This might mean we want to develop or master a new skill, achieve an important goal or win some contest—whatever makes you feel like a winner.

Now when you know which factors contribute to your sense of well-being, let's look at how to incorporate them into your life to make it more rich and meaningful. Nobody says that life should be only flowers and butterflies. But if you want to embody well-being, make sure you often experience pleasure, satisfaction, joy, contentment, peace, and inspiration.

If you don't experience enough positive emotions in your life, stop and think about why.

When it's about your career, you are likely to experience positive emotions only if you use your strengths and talents in your role. Do you?

Think about what makes you happy. Identify people, things, and events that give you pleasure. How can you incorporate some of that into your daily life? Can you meet with a friend more often? Bring some plants into your work environment? Make room in your schedule to attend some joyful event? There's always room for joy and ways to fit it into your routine, if only you decide you won't keep putting these things off into the future...that never quite arrives.

Do you often experience the state of flow? Do you feel you're engaged in your career, or you have hobbies that make you lose yourself and forget about the time?

Although engagement is most often tied to creating, you can experience it through any activity you love—taking part in sports, knitting, gardening, spending time with friends or family, doing a project you're fascinated with.

If you want to slip into the sense of flow and increase your engagement, focus on work, improve your concentration, and minimize distractions, pick the projects that are an interesting challenge to your skills.

Think about your personal interests. Do you make enough time for them? It may be a hobby or a physical activity. When we are stressed and overloaded with work, we easily let these important activities slip away.

Try to reserve enough time for the activities that make you happy and engaged.

Many pieces of research have shown that the most important factor that determines if one is happy and satisfied with their own life is nothing else but connectedness to others. Making and maintaining positive relationships is one of the crucial factors of building a joyful life. All relationships with people fall into this category—your spouse, family, friends, colleagues, neighbors.

Since you probably spend many hours at work, it's important to build good relationships with co-workers. Are your family and friends positive and supportive? Do you enjoy spending time with them? If not, think about why this is so and what you could do to change it. Maybe you need to put more effort and devote more time into strengthening these relationships. Connecting with people takes effort, work, and engagement, but it pays off. On the other hand, keep in mind that you can't do much to change people, so sometimes the ideal solution is to walk away and find support in another place.

Burnout is often the consequence of a lack of sense that our life and work has meaning. We all need to believe that we work and live for some purpose, something bigger than ourselves. Think about meaning in your career. Do you have a sense that you're offering something valuable to humanity? Find meaning in your role or find another purpose closer to your sense of meaning.

When it's about your personal life, certain activities like spending time with your family can bring you a greater sense of meaning. If you lack meaning, engage in activities like playing with kids, volunteering, or even random acts of kindness, and you'll find them very satisfying.

Achievement—this is a tricky one! If you're not devoting enough time to accomplishing your goals and dreams, you won't experience this important part of PERMA model.

But on the other hand, if you are too focused on achievement, you'll slip away from the correct balance and burn out.

The key is in finding and maintaining balance, focusing enough (but not too much) on all aspects of life.

Learn to say "no"

Uttering that little word may be difficult for you. Perhaps you are trying to please everyone and do everything, but until you learn how to say "no," you won't make space for your recovery.

Remind yourself, over and over again, as many times as needed, that you don't have to do everything for everyone, and that your health is now your number one priority. Try not to take on any new responsibilities until you fully recover. That might be challenging, especially if someone needs your help, but you have to learn how to do it politely without hurting others' feelings.

You have to choose wisely which projects and events are worth your effort. At this point, getting rest is more important than accomplishing more, going out, or pleasing anyone. If you don't take care of your health, no one will.

Eliminate the unnecessary

Be merciless about your schedule. Choose only those activities and events that add value to your life, bringing you joy and happiness. Apply the minimalistic approach and choose quality over quantity. There's no place for long working hours, one more project, meaningless conversation with someone who annoys you, sipping coffee and chatting about negative things. You don't have to go to every party and every concert only to not disappoint friends. You don't have to go out when all you want is to stay tucked under a blanket watching Netflix. We don't say you should become a couch potato, but find your balance. Now it's time to recover and you need to pamper yourself.

So everything that can wait—let it wait. There will be plenty of time for fun activities once your energy is back. You can imagine this current state like battery-saving mode on your phone. You need to save energy and not to waste it on anything extra. Spend as little as you can, and only on the basics.

Less is often better

You might not be going to every party, but you'll genuinely enjoy the one you decide to attend.

Maybe you don't have many friends, but those who really love you will be there for you.

You might not talk all the time, but instead of meaningless chatter, you'll enjoy a meaningful conversation.

If you don't work long hours, it doesn't mean you won't be productive. Moreover, it's been discovered that people who work fewer hours achieve more than those who spend more time working.

To cut a long story short, you will lose nothing once you decide to eliminate everything but what is most valuable. Sometimes, less is more.

Practice positive thinking

Yes, easier said than done. When you are tired or lack sleep, it's easy to think negative thoughts. It's a natural response of our amygdala (a part of the brain), responsible for emotional regulation. Positive thinking, on the other hand, requires more energy and effort. How can you do this when you can hardly get out of bed? Burnout makes it super-easy to slip into negative thinking. Moreover, it worsens over time. How can you combat this?

You can learn to think positively. It's a skill, and like any other skill, it can be mastered. There are plenty of techniques you can try out. You can start with affirmations. These are positive statements in the present tense, which declare what you want as if it is already happening. This will help you visualize the future. Visualization is also a great tool because it will make you feel like your dreams are happening for real. You will feel better and believe in what you're doing.

Developing a habit of positive thinking alone is challenging. While recovering from burnout, it might be even harder. But it's imperative, so don't hesitate to get started. Begin with small bites, step by step. Gratitude is one of the most powerful yet easy techniques. Try to take a moment before you get out of bed to think about something nice, something you love, and something you're thankful for. You can also try to close the day this way. Try to remember just one positive thing that happened during, no matter how small. Feel appreciation and gratitude.

Many small moments and little sparks of positivity and joy will group together and build a sense of well-being. Just give it a try and plenty of time.

How meditation can help

Unless you've been living under a rock, chances are you've heard that meditation helps conquer stress. It's absolutely true.

Mindfulness-based stress reduction is a powerful way to recover from burnout, and meditation is its central aspect.

When you are permanently on the go, you can easily disconnect from that voice in your body and soul. You may not be aware of the fact that you're ready to drop, your neck is tense, or you haven't breathed deeper than your upper chest for more than a whole day. Meditation provides an opportunity for you to reconnect with your body.

It also provides you time to observe your thoughts and feelings rather than tackling them. That will calm your busy mind, give you a new perspective, and make more space for productivity and creativity.

If you haven't tried it, give it a chance. It would be best if you meditate before you make your daily to-do list. Those short ten minutes of meditation are simple and should become part your routine like brushing your teeth, not merely another task on your list.

It's extremely simple: you need one burned-out person (check!), a place to sit or lie comfortably and close your eyes, ten minutes in silence, and no distractions.

The easiest way to begin is with a guided program. Put your earplugs in, close your eyes, relax, breathe, and just follow the instructions. Ten minutes a day will do wonders.

It will calm and clear your mind, reduce stress, energize, and rejuvenate you. You'll be better connected with your body and soul, and more aware of your thought and feelings. You'll free your blocked energy and once you recover, all that together will become your shield against exhaustion in the future.

Relax

For people who are always on the go, it might be difficult to slow down. But for finding balance, you need to learn how to bring the body and mind into a state of relaxation. Yet relaxing on command is almost impossible when you are both tired and busy.

When you are in a bad emotional state, it may be very hard just to sit and meditate. You may start with simple breathing exercises to calm the nervous system. To begin with, or to prepare for meditation practice, breathe mindfully—inhale slowly through your nose, then slowly exhale as if you were breathing out through a straw.

Practicing yoga will also help you quickly chill out.

If you are still searching for a kind of conscious rest that will suit you the best, try out massage and acupuncture. All of those techniques are proven to help in relaxation and recovery from extreme fatigue.

Do nothing, regularly

Getting massages, going to a spa, doing aromatherapy, going to yoga, and lying on your acupuncturist's table are all beneficial. All these little steps will accumulate and bring you up from your drained state. But sometimes, the best thing you can do for yourself, is nothing.

For constantly wired overachievers, the concept of doing nothing might seem nebulous. So if you have to do something, here are some suggestions on the ways you can "do nothing":

- Take a nap.
- Lie on the ground, look at the sky, and focus on your breathing.
- Sit beside a large body of water and just look at it for a while.
- Take a luxurious salt or bubble bath.
- Blow soap bubbles and watch them float away.

Your urge to always be busy doing something has slipped out of control. It's drained you. Now, when you are trying to turn the process in the opposite direction, it's crucial to actually do the opposite, which is *nothing*.

Make room for play and laughter

Laughter is a precious cure for almost everything. If you feel you lack joy and play, you surely do. That's the part that we lose sight of the easiest. Our culture appreciates being serious, always busy, and tired. Being cheerful, optimistic, and smiling too often is labeled as being silly and immature.

If you barely wake up and already can't wait the day to come to an end, life is not funny at all. If you take everything too seriously, life can seem hard and an all-or-nothing kind of choice.

Decide to find laughter, play, and joy again.

Make time for it. Do whatever is needed to prioritize it. Watch a comedy, meet with a humorous friend, do more of what makes you playful and cheerful. There must be something that tickles your funny bone. Do more of it. This could be your path away from exhaustion.

How to Prevent Burnout in the Future

Evaluate burnout potential in your life

How is your physical condition? Are you strong enough to stand any amount of long-term stress, or do you have to be careful about the amount of stress you tolerate? Do you become easily tired or sick?

Consider your career or work situation

Do you work at the job you love? Do you have all of the ability you need to succeed? Are you valued and do you work in a supportive environment? Do you feel overworked? Do you have to choose between long hours at work and time with your family? Are you paid enough?

Assess your relationships

Is your family a warm, loving, and supportive one, or do you feel more resentment and unhappiness thinking about them? Are you happy with your spouse, if you have one? Do you have supportive close friends you can turn to?

Consider the season

Is there a time of year when you are more overloaded and have increased responsibilities?

Evaluate your life in general

Is it delightful, manageable, stressful, or unbearable? Is there burnout knocking on your door?

Get enough rest

It's not enough to go on vacation once a year. Everyone needs daily rest reserved for relaxation and recharging, a weekly rest time (two days off), and a vacation when you get away from your work environment. To prevent yourself from getting to the edge of exhaustion, afford yourself enough quality sleep at night. That's a priority and there shouldn't be any compromise.

Take care of yourself

You are irreplaceable only to yourself. Everybody else could somehow find a way to move on without you. Your work can function without you. Even your family can exist without you. The world would move on with or without you. It sounds cruel, but it's true.

Taking care of yourself is not selfish. You can't give what you don't have. In other words, if you are not good to yourself, you won't be good for anyone else. Sleep enough, eat well, exercise regularly. Stay hydrated and learn how to breathe. Afford yourself tiny treats and satisfactions.

Set aside one day a week for unplugging

If you are constantly available, that's adding to your stress. You can't be absolutely focused when you can be interrupted at anytime. Decide to limit your screen time, like with children, and your "available" time. Limit all of your time online. Check email only once or twice a day. Turn off your phone while you are with family or friends. Leave it on silent mode, in another room. Turn off your laptop while it's charging. Set aside one day a week when you'll stay offline for the whole day. That will help you regularly check in with yourself and stay connected and grounded.

Connect, grow your relationships, and get support

If you often feel lonely and that you have no one to turn to, it's time to find new friends or reconnect with old ones. Put in the effort in your relationships with family and friends. Loneliness is not good for your happiness, but it's also contributing to your exhaustion. Our positive relationships keep us on the surface and make life seem worth living, even if the interactions are not always profound.

Exercise

Don't wait to feel completely drained. Do something about your physical activity today. Go for a walk. Sign up for yoga classes or even rumba, samba, pilates, anything, as long as it makes you happy and keeps you moving. Regularly practicing physical exercise might save you from slipping into burnout. It may also help in recovery, but it's far easier to start while you still have some energy in you.

Learn to meditate and to be mindful

If you still haven't tried, it's time to learn how to meditate. You don't need a lot of theoretical knowledge. It's more about practice. You'll master it by sitting, breathing, and doing nothing. Find a guided program for beginners, ten free minutes, and give it a try.

Being mindful is one of the most precious gifts you could give yourself. This means being aware of the life happening around you. Start with small exercises, not longer than a few minutes. For instance, you can try to be completely present and aware of sensations while you are drinking a glass of water, or while you're doing the dishes. Put the effort into adopting a mindful approach to life and it will be deeply rewarding.

Find a creative outlet

Being too achievement-focused makes you rigid, and you may lack creativity and flexibility. That's why it's important to find some way to express yourself through creativity or to revive an old hobby. Creativity lowers stress levels, increases feelings of joy, and heightens the connection with yourself. No matter which type of creative activity you choose, it will keep you engaged and motivated.

Improve your self-esteem

Self-efficacy is believing that you have the ability to accomplish your goals and tasks. People who have a higher level of self-esteem believe they can cope with whatever life throws at them. They experience less stress in challenging situations. You can efficiently build self-efficacy through accomplishment. When you achieve one goal, you ask yourself what else you can achieve. This expands your comfort zone and boosts your self-esteem because you see how you can cope with everything.

Boost positive emotions

Little positive things will accumulate to make you feel happy and resilient to stress. That is the best protection you can build against burnout. Start noticing good things around you—what someone has done well, what you can be grateful for, what you have done right. Notice everything that can make you smile—from new shoes to beautiful flowers to huge achievements. All of that is part of life, and everything is worth your attention. Don't let yourself shrink to one aspect of life and then focus all of your effort on all-or-nothing. Do everything you can for your mental hygiene, adopt a positive mindset, and make yourself feel good as much and as often as possible.

Conclusion

You can compare yourself to your cell phone. When your battery is close to empty, it signals you. You can plug in the charger or ignore the signals. If you decide to ignore them, it will turn off. If you choose to charge the battery, you will need to put the phone aside and let it recharge. If it has too little time to do so, it won't be fully charged, and the battery will soon be empty again.

Don't let yourself empty the whole of your battery and then shut down. Be kind to yourself and recharge your energy in time so you don't have to live in "battery-saver" mode.

Now you know how to recognize if you are already on the road to exhaustion. The best you can do is to stop, recharge, and then change your path. Once you are recovered, prevent it from happening again in the future. Create a strong net to hold you and keep yourself from falling into this state again.